Oleg Petrović
Nebojša Sindik

Clinical Use of Continuous Epidural Analgesia in Vaginal Deliveries

Oleg Petrović
Nebojša Sindik

Clinical Use of Continuous Epidural Analgesia in Vaginal Deliveries

Indications, Clinical Use, Drugs, Benefits and Complications

LAP LAMBERT Academic Publishing

Impressum / Imprint

Bibliografische Information der Deutschen Nationalbibliothek: Die Deutsche Nationalbibliothek verzeichnet diese Publikation in der Deutschen Nationalbibliografie; detaillierte bibliografische Daten sind im Internet über http://dnb.d-nb.de abrufbar. Alle in diesem Buch genannten Marken und Produktnamen unterliegen warenzeichen-, marken- oder patentrechtlichem Schutz bzw. sind Warenzeichen oder eingetragene Warenzeichen der jeweiligen Inhaber. Die Wiedergabe von Marken, Produktnamen, Gebrauchsnamen, Handelsnamen, Warenbezeichnungen u.s.w. in diesem Werk berechtigt auch ohne besondere Kennzeichnung nicht zu der Annahme, dass solche Namen im Sinne der Warenzeichen- und Markenschutzgesetzgebung als frei zu betrachten wären und daher von jedermann benutzt werden dürften.

Bibliographic information published by the Deutsche Nationalbibliothek: The Deutsche Nationalbibliothek lists this publication in the Deutsche Nationalbibliografie; detailed bibliographic data are available in the Internet at http://dnb.d-nb.de. Any brand names and product names mentioned in this book are subject to trademark, brand or patent protection and are trademarks or registered trademarks of their respective holders. The use of brand names, product names, common names, trade names, product descriptions etc. even without a particular marking in this works is in no way to be construed to mean that such names may be regarded as unrestricted in respect of trademark and brand protection legislation and could thus be used by anyone.

Coverbild / Cover image: www.ingimage.com

Verlag / Publisher:
LAP LAMBERT Academic Publishing
ist ein Imprint der / is a trademark of
OmniScriptum GmbH & Co. KG
Heinrich-Böcking-Str. 6-8, 66121 Saarbrücken, Deutschland / Germany
Email: info@lap-publishing.com

Herstellung: siehe letzte Seite /
Printed at: see last page
ISBN: 978-3-659-50439-6

Zugl. / Approved by: Rijeka, University of Rijeka, Diss., 2012

ABSTRACT

The primary objectives of this 2-year clinical study were to test the impact of continuous epidural analgesia (EA) on the duration of the first and the second stage of labour, and on the incidence of operative deliveries in the group of singleton pregnancies at 35-41 weeks with fetus in cephalic presentation.

A total of 2,126 patients and their vaginal deliveries at the Department of Gyn/Ob, University Hospital Center in Rijeka were analysed. In the group with EA (n=1,083) the median values of duration of the first and the second stage of delivery were significantly longer than in the control group. Vacuum extractions and caesarean sections were significantly more represented in deliveries with EA. There were no statistically significant differences between the groups for any variable of neonatal outcome.

Continuous EA has been proven as safe and it should be considered the method of first choice for reliable delivery analgesia. However, its application may significantly prolong both delivery stages and increase the number of operative deliveries, particularly caesarean sections. The reasons lie in the uncritical use of regional analgesia and strict application of classical obstetric criteria. Therefore, the authors recommend an individualized approach for each parturient woman in order to reduce the unfavourable effects of EA.

TABLE OF CONTENTS

CHAPTER I: BIRTH PAIN AND METHODS OF ANALGESIA

CHAPTER II: OBJECTIVES OF THE STUDY

CHAPTER III: STUDY POPULATION AND METHODS

CHAPTER IV: RESULTS OF THE STUDY

CHAPTER V: DISCUSSION AND REFERENCES

LIST OF FIGURES

LIST OF TABLES

CHAPTER I: BIRTH PAIN AND METHODS OF ANALGESIA

Introduction – brief history of birth pain

From Roman period onwards during centuries that followed throughout the European continent nothing was done to facilitate the birth pain to women in labour. Traditionally, physicians of that time were not actively dealing with labour pain, despite the fact that many historical manuscripts of early civilizations described the term of birth pain and methods for its moderations. Ancient Chinese manuscripts describe the use of opiates and narcotics as means for relieving pain during the labour. Helen of Troy knew how to prepare a medicine out of mix of herbs which was used to erase the labour pain from the memory. Women from the Apache tribe had a tradition of hanging from the tree during the labour tied with leather strap under their underarms, while the husband pushed with all his strength the fundus of the uterus. In the Pacific islands of Pago, generations of women were giving birth kneeling while man was standing behind the woman, pushing her back (1, 2).

Until the 19th century analgesia was not used during the labour. Attitudes towards birth pain begin to change when the School of Midwifery was established in Edinburgh at 1726, which improved the status of women making their lifes more valauble and giving rise to desire to help a woman durin labour (3).

On October 4th 1847, James Simpson first used the ether anaesthesia during vaginal delivery, but was attacked by Scottish Calvinists who referred to quote written in Bible: *"I will greatly multiply your pain in childbirth, in pain you will bring forth children"*. But, Simpson answered to his opponents that *God* narcotized Adam to take out his rib making him the first anesthesiologist (*"Anesthesia is the art of God"*). Sir James Clark revealed, Queen Victoria's obstetrician, informed Simpson in 1853 by letter that a physician John Snow, pioneer in anesthesiology, used chloroform while the Queen was giving birth to her eighth child, prince Leopold (4). Possible harmful effects of chloroform and ether on uterine activity were detected during relatively early stages of their use. John Snow wrote that in some earlier cases during which chloroform was used, uterine contractions were so weakened that forceps had to be applied to complete delivery.

A mixture of nitrous oxide and oxygen was for the first time used in 1880 in St. Petersburg, to facilitate the delivery of 25 childbearing women. Since 1900 when assistant Oscar Kreis first used the spinal block as an analgesic during labour at *Women's hospital* in Basel, the regional techniques for pain management increasingly showed all their advantages. Caudal analgesia in decreasing labour pain was first introduced by Walter Stoeckel in 1909 (1). But it was not notedly used until 1936 when Charles Odom, a surgeon in *Humanitarian Hospital* in Louisiana, first reported about the use of lumbar epidural anesthesia during the caesarean section (5). George Pitkin used the term of *controlled spinal anesthesia* for the first time in 1928 (3). By describing the technique, precautions and security measures, he made the spinal anesthesia during labour popular in the United States of America (USA). In 1933, Cleland was the first who realized that dysfunctional contractions were normalized after a successful analgesia. *Demerol*, a synthetic substitute for morphine, was introduced into obstetric practice in 1938. Lumbar epidural block was used for the first time during a labour in 1941 in the United States of America (USA) (6). Catheterization techniques for continuous epidural analgesia were described in 1949 by Curbelo from Cuba, and the same year, Flowers et al. introduced them into obstetrics. Phillip Bromage, who had an important role in popularization of this technique, wrote that continuous epidural analgesia is not a technique for anesthesiologists who only occasionally deal with it, because it requires a certain degree of skills and decision that probably can not be achieved without special training and experience (3).

The beginnings of regional analgesia in the Republic of Croatia started in Zagreb and Rijeka during 1977, while in Slovenia regional analgesia was used for the first time in 1982 in capital city of Ljubljana (7, 8).

Birth pain

Labour is a natural, physiological process which is subject to physical rules and representing the expulsion of fetus to the external environment through the birth canal with the help of uterine contractions. Labour is carried on according to the mechanism of labour, which is defined as a set of interaction effects between the main elements of labour. It begins with the appearance of regular uterine contractions (or rupture of membranes) and ends with the baby, as well as placenta and fetal membranes being born. From the clinical point of view, four stages of labour can be recognised.

The first stage of labour (= *cervical dilation stage*) starts with the appearance of regular preparatory contractions (lat. *Dolores preparantes*) whose occurrence interval shortens from 30 minutes to 3-4 minutes and lasts for 30 seconds. Throughout 6-14 hours of duration, of which about 9 hours are latent phase, and the remaining 3-5 hours are active phase, a progressive shortening of the cervix occurs. Vaginal portion of the cervix is centered in a guiding line of the birth canal while the cervical opening expands. Active management of the first stage of labour involves amniotomy and stimulation of uterine contractions. The first stage of labour ends by a complete cervical dilation up to 10 cm.

The second stage of labour (= *fetal expulsion stage)* starts after a complete dilation of the cervical opening, accompanied by a rupture of membranes. It lasts from 30 minutes to 2 hours. Uterine contractions (lat. *Dolores ad partum*) occur frequently, every 2-3 minutes and last up to 60 seconds. During that time lowering, flexion and rotation of the fetal head occurs. Head, pressuring the soft parts of the birth canal and the last part of the colon,

7

causes reflexive activation of so called *abdominal prelum* which increases the force of uterine contractions three to four-fold and pushes the fetal head to exit the pelvis.

Pain caused by labour contractions represents a great problem for many childbearing women. Intensity of experienced pain, a result of interaction of neurophysiological, psychological and sociocultural factors, varies from person to person. It is estimated that about 5% of childbearing women do not ask for any type of analgesia, and 15% of women cooperate poorly or do not cooperate at all due to unsupportable pain during delivery (lat. *Dolorem sedare divinum opus est*). There are two types of a delivery pain: visceral and somatic pain (9, 10). In different phases of delivery, painful impulses are transmitted through neural pathways to the different levels of the spinal cord.

During the first stage of labour, rhythmic contractions of the uterus and ensuing dilation of the cervix oppening cause the occurrence of delivery pain. This type of pain is known as visceral and is transmitted through alpha A and visceral C fibres coming out of the uterine body. These enter the ventral radices of 10th, 11th and 12th thoracic and 1st lumbar segment of the spinal cord through the hypogastric plexus, and lumbar and thoracic segment of the sympathetic chain component (Figure 1). Pain occurs only if the intrauterine pressure exceeds the threshold of 25 mmHg. It is transmitted slowly and hardly localized in the lower abdomen area i.e. lumbosacral area (4, 11).

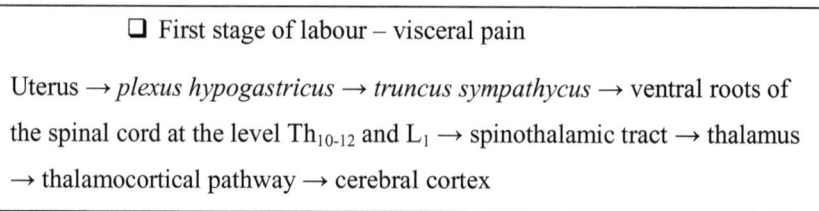

Figure 1. Birth pain in the first stage of delivery

In the second stage of delivery, pain occurs due to cervix dilation, and dilation of the pelvic floor, combined with the pressure of the fetal head on vaginal wall and perineum. Painful impulses are transmitted through A fibres along *n. pudendus* to the 2nd, 3rd and 4th sacral spinal cord segments (Figure 2). By its nature, the pain is somatic, strong and can be precisely localized (9, 10). Visceral and somatic pain travels through spinothalamic tract to thalamus and then by thalamocortical pathway to cerebral cortex. Stress caused by pain is followed by a series of hormonal, hemodynamic, respiratory, metabolic and

---

❑ Second stage of labour - somatic pain

Pelvic floor → *nn.pudendi* → ventral roots of the spinal cord at the level S_{2-4} → spinothalamic tract → thalamus → thalamocortical radiations → cerebral cortex

---

Figure 2. Birth pain in the second stage of delivery

psychological changes that influence the progress of labour and the state of fetus. The release of catecholamines, cortisol and adrenocorticotropic hormone (ACTH) is increased while the body's need for oxygen grows. Increased catecholamine concentrations in the blood of women during labour reduce uterine and placental blood flow and constrict umbilical cord vessels, which can lead to hypoxia and acidosis (15). Pathophysiological processes, activated as a response to pain, enhance existing hyperventilation caused by progesterone. During hyperventilation, the partial pressure of carbon dioxide (pCO_2) decreases and alkalosis occurs. After an uterine contraction, due to hypocapnia, a transitory hypoventilation occurs, reducing the partial pressure of oxygen in arterial blood. Decrease of pO_2 in mother's blood under 9.3 kPa significantly affects the fetus oxygenation which results in subsequent fetal acidosis. Cardiac output increases the rate of 15-20% at the beginning and 150% at the end of delivery. Increase of the cardiac pressure up to 50% occurs due to the redistribution of uterine blood flow towards the maternal circulation and due to increased sympathetic activity activated by pain. Therefore, the increase in blood pressure is particularly dangerous for pregnant women who suffer from heart disease, hypertension and pre-eclampsia.

Every childbearing woman deals with uterine contractions and pain during vaginal delivery. Fear felt by woman may further stimulate spasm of the lower uterine segment (LUS) commonly exacerbating the pain. This in turn increases the sense of fear and uncertainty regarding perinatal outcome. The described "vicious circle" results in a poor collaboration of the childbearing woman, her distrust and impatience and very often with prolongation or complete slowdown of delivery. The aforementioned situation often requires employment of adequate obstetric surgeries. Therefore, reduction or elimination of the labour pain imposes as a logical and preventive solution (12, 13).

The arising question is how to safely help the woman and suppress the pain during delivery while jeopardizing neither the mother nor the baby. Mother and the baby are mutually connected that is separated by the semipermeable placental membrane allowing analgesics, sedatives and anesthetics given to mother to be transferred into the fetal circulation (14).

Methods of obstetric analgesia

All the different methods to relieve or eliminate labour pains that have been and are still used in modern obstetrics, can be divided into two basic groups:

- non-pharmacological: proper breathing techniques, psycho prophylaxis, massage, hypnosis, hydrotherapy, audio-analgesia, transcutaneous electrical nerve neurostimulation (TENS), acupuncture (16);
- pharmacological:

- o systematic analgesic drugs, inhalation anesthetics, tranquilizers and sedatives (dosage of parenterally introduced analgesics is limited due to the risk of sedation and respiratory insufficiency of mother and fetus) (17);
- o nerve block techniques: peripheral (paracervical and pudendal block) and central (caudal, epidural, spinal and combined block) (18).

Psychological methods for pain reduction can be performed in individual or group therapy within courses for preparing pregnant women or physical exercises for pregnant women.

Hypnosis causes intense relaxation and represents a state of severe suggestibility, thanks to which the childbearing woman accepts the analgesia suggestions. Hypnosis does not provoke the release of endorphins, but through suggestive content activates frontal cortex and limbic system that inhibits the transmission of pain impulses from the thalamus to the cortex. With the support of their closest, primarily spouses or partners, a childbearing woman additionally gains the needed sense of security and becomes relaxed, all of which reduce fear, tension and pain.

Transcutaneous electrical nerve neurostimulation (TENS) implies electrical stimulation of nerve endings in the skin and stimulation of A and C nerve fibres, thus preventing pain to reach the higher levels of the nervous system.

Acupuncture is a method of stimulating skin points rich of nerve endings, thus activating pain-relieving mechanisms situated in the spinal cord. The above described technique, when used, involves the humoral factors in the mechanism of analgesia, through hypothalamic-pituitary axis where it stimulates the release of beta-endorphins.

Paracervical block represents a local anesthetic infiltration in the paracervical tissue. The aforementioned block stops the transmission of pain impulses from uterine cervix, the lowest region of the uterus through the inferior hypogastric plexus (lat. *Plexus hypogastricus inferior*) located in loose connective tissue between uterosacral ligaments and in close connection with the uterine artery and venous plexus, ureter, the lower uterine segment and fetus itself. It is applied in the first stage of labour. *Bupivacaine* 0.25 – 0.125% is used for anesthesia. The volume of 10 mL should be divided into two injection sites i.e. at "4 and 5 hours" on right, and at "7 and 8 hours" on left. Before injecting the local anesthetics all the necessary precautions should be taken to avoid accidental intravascular injection or injection to the baby.

During pudendal block, the obstetrician injects 1% of *Lidocaine* through the vaginal wall with the intention of pudendal nerve blocking. Paracervical block in the first stage as well as pudendal and caudal blocks in the second stage of labour, today are very rarely applied.

Caudal block is best suitable for analgesia in the second stage of labour. Through the sacral hiatus (lat. *Hiatus sacralis)* 20 ml of 2% *Lidocaine* is injected in the sacral canal. It is important to take all precautionary measures as well as for pudendal block due to possible complications.

Epidural analgesia provides the most comprehensive analgesia, having many advantages in comparison to parenteral analgesia (by giving opiates) and inhalation analgesic techniques (19, 20). In relation to the spinal block, the effects of analgesia occur more slowly, but last longer, with fewer adverse effects on placental hemodynamics while the muscular block is also significantly weaker. The parturient woman is calm and cooperative throughout the delivery and mobilizes much faster after delivery than after the use of opioids and general anesthesia. In some cases, epidural analgesia may favorably influence the incoordinated uterine activity. Analgesia is achieved by injecting the anesthetics in the epidural space. Concentrations of local anesthetics in maternal and fetal plasma are very low and do not influence adversely on the blood flow through the umbilical cord, Apgar scores and neurological examination results (21, 22). Moreover, by interrupting nerve impulse transmission pathways from peripheral pain receptors and denervation of the core of adrenal glands, epidural analgesia can increase uteroplacental blood flow and thus improve the state of mother and fetus. It can be used as an intermittent, continuous, spinal-epidural analgesia and analgesia controlled by the patient herself (23).

Due to the lack of intermittent epidural injection is impossible to determine the concentration of anesthetics required, and as a consequence, pain and/or motoric block may reappear and prolong the second stage of labour or also stop the delivery (24). Such complication can be prevented by administration of repetitive doses which are 75-100% of the initial dose of medicine.

Continuous epidural analgesia is also more efficient since there is no discontinuity of analgesic activity. It can be achieved by giving lower concentrations of anesthetics so even the motor block appears more rarely. It meets the various conditions required during spontaneous or instrumental vaginal delivery and caesarean section. However, perineal analgesia in the second stage of labour is insufficient if the anticipated duration of delivery is longer than two hours. Positioning of an epidural catheter in pregnancy is often difficult due to the lumbar lordosis and insufficient leg flexion of the childbearing woman, tissue edema, and lack of cooperation with the childbearing woman. The epidural space volume decreases for about 40%, and together with lumbar hyperlordosis enhances the spread of local anesthetics toward the head while the muscular block also reduces the diffusion of the of anesthetics toward caudal. The risk of needle or a catheter vascular puncture is 10-12% greater in comparison to 1% at patients that are not pregnant. Epidural veins blood flow during pregnancy is significantly higher and accidental application of local anesthetics into a vein leads to its concentration upsurge in the brain and in the heart. Cerebrospinal fluid pressure in the lumbar epidural space is increased and further rises during the uterine contractions, providing an increased risk of the dural puncture. In childbearing women the puncture should be performed between contractions, at the midline and at the height of L2/L3 and L3/L4, where the epidural space is widest (width varies from 5 to 8 mm), ensuring a very small possibility of accidental puncture of epidural veins due to their more lateral position. Epidural space is identified by loss of resistance to air or saline, so before introducing anestetics an aspiration must be used to determine that the needle peak is not accidentally in a vein or spinal space (25-27). Contraindications to the use of epidural analgesia during labour as an invasive procedure limit its non-selective use in all childbearing women. Thus, epidural analgesia is not applied to childbearing women who do not want to relieve delivery pain regardless of the existence of some of the medical indications, in those suffering from diseases of the central nervous system (multiple sclerosis, a condition of increased intracranial pressure due to a tumor or hemorrhage), those with the inflammatory process in the puncture area or greater deformation of the lumbar spine, those who suffer from sepsis or are in the (pre)shock state called hypovolemia, who take anticoagulant therapy or show signs of bleeding diathesis (28). Insufficient obstetric and anesthesiological team education is one of the classic contraindications for introduction of epidural analgesia during labour (29). Clinical chorioamnionitis and fever are not contraindications, but in such cases a preventive administration of antibiotics is recommended (4). There will be fewer complications if the aforementioned contraindications are considered. The most frequent complications are post-dural puncture headache due to cerebrospinal fluid leakage, intracranial pressure decrease and cerebral vasodilatation in accidental dura mater puncture (30-34), postpartum low back pain (35), urinary retention as a consequence of prolonged effects of local analgesics (36, 37), hypotension in pregnant woman (systolic blood pressure <100 mmHg or a decrease of systolic blood pressure > 25% in comparison with the blood pressure prior to analgesia) due to accompanying sympathetic block (9, 29, 38) and fever ≥ 38°C as a reaction to a foreign body (catheter) (39-41). Convulsions or cardiovascular collapse occur rarely as a consequence of an accidental intravenous administration of anesthetics, systematic toxic reaction to an administered medication or a complete spinal anesthesia during the dura mater lesion and subarachnoid injection of inadequate quantity of anesthetics (29, 42).

Combined spinal and epidural anaesthesia as a form of analgesia is also used during delivery, although it is best suited for caesarean section where a good muscular relaxation is required. Analgesics are injected through a needle into the spinal subarachnoid space thus achieving an instantaneous analgesia, and then an epidural catheter is introduced ensuring the continuing epidural analgesia (43-50).

A newer version of continuous epidural analgesia is patient-controlled epidural analgesia (PCEA) where woman during labour has the possibility to actively control the intensity of analgesia within certain limits (51-55). Possibility of self-control of birth pain makes her mentally more stable, more satisfied of more willing to cooperate (56, 57).

Selection of local anesthetics for analgesia is based on their analgesic effects and duration, placental transfer, toxicity and the level of motor block. Concentration of anesthetics in fetal plasma is the result of total administered dose of local anesthetics, their absorption into the blood vessels, of local anesthetic binding to mother's plasma proteins and of the fetus and of dissociation constants of anesthetics themselves. Unionised fraction of local anesthetics easily passes through the placental membrane, while the binding to plasma proteins reduce its "passage" through the placenta. Due to the local vasodilatory effect and possible entrance of local anesthetics into the circulation, adrenaline in concentration 1: 200,000 should be added.

Bupivacaine is the best analgesic choice as it has the best characteristics needed for the obstetric analgesia. About 95% of the drug binds to proteins, its action is longer than 90 minutes and there is no tachyphylaxis thus achieving a moderate sensory and motor block. Cardiotoxicity is a side effect of *Bupivacaine*, so the total dose should not exceed 150 mg in a single injection or a maximum of 300 mg during 10 hours, which is why concentrations higher than 0.5% are not used. In comparison with *Bupivacaine*, *Chirocaine (Levobupivacaine)* is somehow less cardiotoxic and neurotoxic. *Ropivacaine* has a similar chemical structure than *Bupivacaine* (58). It causes a local vasoconstriction thus offsetting the weaker affinity for proteins so the duration of block is slightly shorter than that of *Bupivacaine*. Motor block is weaker which provides it with a certain advantage over the *Bupivacaine* (59). By adding opioids, particularly highly lipophilic ones like *Fentanyl* and *Sufentanyl*, the quality of analgesic block raises, the appearance of incomplete block decreases thus resulting in enhanced block of sacral nerve radices. Administration of lower concentration of local anesthetics reduces the motor block and enables a more natural force of pushing.

For a continuous epidural analgesia in obstetrics a 0.125% solution of *Bupivacaine* or a 0.125 % solution *Chirocaine* with 2.5 µg *Fentanyl* per milliliter of infusion (2-4 µg of *Fentanyl* per milliliter of epidural infusion is allowed) are used. Instead of *Fentanyl*, with the same concentration of *Bupivacaine* or *Chirocaine* per milliliter of epidural analgesia, 0.5 µg of *Sufentanyl* can be added (60-63).

Pain that occurs during delivery has been recognized as a cause of the increased number of delivery delays and medical interventions. Epidural analgesia has been introduced in the obstetric practice precisely in order to eliminate or reduce the delivery pain that occurs due to uterine contractions, cervical dilation and distension of perineal tissue during the first and the second stage of labor. Several authors reported on its analgesic effects that facilitates cervix dilation and enables painless descent of the fetal head to the bottom of the birth canal, thus accelerating the progress of labour in medically induced cases (64-66). Use of epidural analgesia has significantly increased in the world over the last 10 years, and by introducing the aforementioned method on request it has become common in delivery rooms around the world (9, 16, 67-71). It is estimated that an average of 25-30% of childbearing women in the UK and the USA use this method of analgesia, while in some centers that percentage exceeds even 50%, mostly being used in deliveries of primiparous women (67, 72-74).

In Croatia, so far there is no reliable clinical reports about usage of continuous epidural analgesia in obstetric practice, nor were systematically investigated the advantages of its use in labour in relation to the possible disadvantages. Namely, epidural analgesia changes the dynamics of delivery process as no other method of analgesia, by speeding up or slowing down some of its phases (11, 38, 68, 75). The result is easier cervical dilation, but also weakened or completely eliminated physiological reflex mechanisms that normally enhance uterine contractions at pressure of the fetus head on the pelvic floor, so there is a possibility of extending, particularly the second stage of labour as well as that the final stage of delivery with the adverse effects on perinatal outcome (76-78). Moreover, the literature showed up several reports that warn of an increased incidence of operative deliveries related to the use of epidural analgesia (79-83). In such conditions it becomes questionable whether one should fully adhere to the criteria of classical obstetrics in conducting the second stage of labor as well as the final stage of delivery. There are not enough well-documented studies or unique conclusions in literature about that. Moreover, despite the proven benefits, since the beginning of epidural analgesia use, its overall effects on the progress of labour are one of many controversial topics among obstetricians (84). While everyone agrees that epidural analgesia reduces the intensity of the birth pain, everything else is still a subject of a lively debate (85). Particularly controversial are the results of the research related to the operative or instrumental deliveries. Some authors in their papers were often unilaterally using different selection criteria in selection of a group of respondents (primiparous and multiparous), analysed various techniques of epidural analgesia, various drugs and doses of drugs and all this on relatively small samples (86-91). Thus is not surprising that an often cited conclusion is a need for further research for a better understanding of complex effects of the epidural analgesia on the course and outcome of labour (4, 87).

There is no possibility of using experimental models in laboratory conditions for researching the influence of epidural analgesia on entire course and outcome of labour as well as on the perinatal outcome, so a well-planned clinical study with a sufficient number of patients in strictly defined groups and implementation of appropriate scientific methods is the only way to acquire the relevant facts on using the aforementioned analgesic methods in vaginal deliveries. Our hypothesis is that the uncritical use of continuous epidural analgesia in the second stage of labor and particularly in the final stage of labor, and a strict routine use of prevailing classical criteria for conducting vaginal deliveries are the main causes of increased frequency of operative deliveries. Taking into account the reports of numerous worlds' renowned authors about favourable, but also about adverse effects of epidural analgesia on the vaginal delivery outcomes, we decided to retrospectively analyse the influence of continuous epidural analgesia on increased frequency of operative deliveries, as exactly this fact, like no other, could adversly affect the attitude of obstetricians towards an epidural analgesia and diminish its well-deserved popularity.

CHAPTER II: OBJECTIVES OF THE STUDY

Objectives of the study

The primary objective of this study was to examine the effects of continuous epidural analgesia on duration of the active phase of the first stage of labor and the course of the second stage, with particular emphasis on operative termination of deliveries. Secondary objectives of this study was to determine the most common indications for using the continuous epidural analgesia in labour, the frequency and importance of certain specific intrapartum and postpartum complications, the influence of epidural analgesia on the neonatal outcome, and to provide practical recommendations for conducting vaginal deliveries under epidural analgesia.

CHAPTER III: STUDY POPULATION AND METHODS

Study population

A clinical study included more than 1,000 singleton vaginal deliveries of at least 35 weeks of gestation during which continuous epidural analgesia (EPA) has been applied. This study was performed during a 2-year period, from January 1, 2009 to December 31, 2010 at University Hospital Center Rijeka, Department of Gynecology and Obstetrics – Perinatal Unit. All cases that required urgent operative termination of pregnancy were excluded from this study. After all the examinees were explained the advantages and possible complications that may occur during procedure in a comprehensible way, they all had signed their informed consent for the aforementioned medical intervention. This study was approved by the University Hospital Center Rijeka Ethics Committee.

Control group included pregnant women and deliveries who were next in line after the examinees, according to the ordinal number delivery protocol (document in which all deliveries are chronologically recorded in one calendar year). Patients in control group were of the same or similar age, constitutional characteristics, parity, duration of pregnancy and obstetric findings and did not differ regarding the complications in pregnancy (for example, premature rupture of membranes, diabetes, hypertensive disorders, etc.). If the next childbearing women from the list also gave birth under the epidural analgesia, she was included in the control group as the next in line. A special subgroup among the examined vaginal deliveries was formed of those cases in which the second stage of labour was actively conducted while the epidural analgesia was discontinuated or significantly reduced in the final stage of delivery (at cervical dilation of 8-10 cm).

Methods

The study is based on a retrospective review of data from carefully registered and managed medical records (medical histories, partograms and anaesthesiology records) and statistical analysis of relevant indicators: age, parity, height, weight and body mass index of childbearing women, gestational age, type of delivery onset (contractions, premature rupture of membranes, labour induction), labour duration (independently the first and the second stage of labour), indication for giving epidural analgesia, mode of deliveries (spontaneous delivery, vacuum extraction, caesarean section), intrapartum epidural analgesia complications and perinatal outcomes. We considered the appearance of regular contractions every 10 minutes or leakage of amniotic fluid as the onset of delivery. Appearance of variable and/or late decelerations, fetal bradycardia and/or tachycardia and silent type of curve were considered pathologic cardiotocographic findings. Perinatal outcome was rated based on the following data: sex, birth weight, distribution frequency of Apgar scores <7 in the 5th minute after delivery, pH value of fetal and / or arterial umbilical blood <7.20 and early neonatal morbidity and mortality. If the delivery was completed operatively, the indications listed in the medical records were analysed. The postpartum course and particular complications that occurred by using the continuous epidural analgesia (fever, allergic reaction, hypotension, urinary retention, post puncture headache, complete spinal anesthesia) were also observed.

Epidural catheter was introduced in the delivery room according to our protocol for catheter introduction during the delivery. The adequate preparation of a childbearing woman in order to prevent intrapartum epidural analgesia complications was required in all cases. It consisted of a thorough anamnesis for possible drug allergies, coagulopathy, neurological disorders, hypotonia, spinal deformities and prior spinal surgery as well as inflammatory processes at the puncture points, physical examination, blood pressure and pulse measurement of a childbearing woman and the introduction of an intravenous path and hydration with 500-1000 mL of crystalloid solution, with continuous electronic fetal heart monitoring. Before the puncture itself, a puncture point was determined with childbearing woman in side position (Figure 3a) or while sitting afterwards disinfection and skin protection was done using sterile compresses (Figure 3b). Then infiltration of the back skin with 1% *Xylocaine* followed, and the epidural space was identified by use of the needle (Figure 4).

Puncture point is at the level of L2/L3 or L3/L4 to enable the epidural block during the first stage of labour to include the lower thoracic and upper lumbar segments of the spinal cord. Then the catheter was introduced through a needle into the epidural space (Figure 5), the top of which was positioned 2-3 cm cranially. Through the catheter a test dose of 2-3 mL of 2% *Lidocaine* was injected (92).

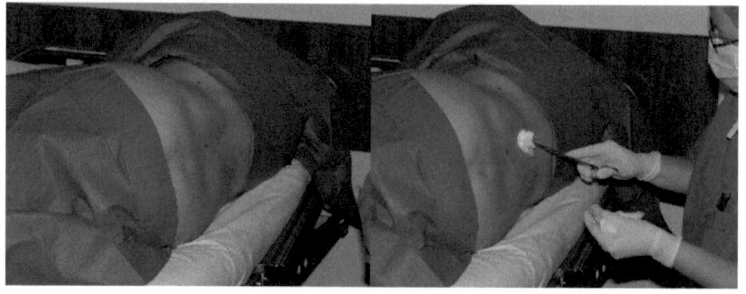

Figure 3. Determining puncture point with childbearing woman
in side position (a) and skin disinfection (b)

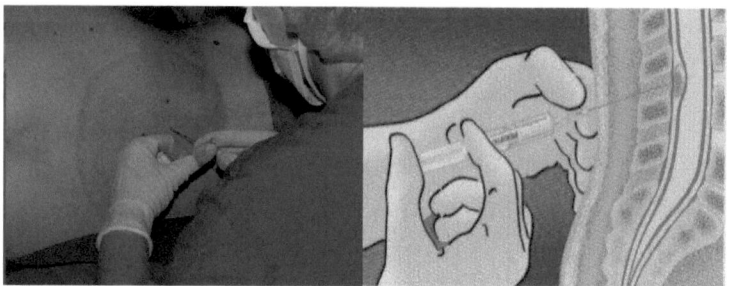

Figure 4. Identification of epidural area

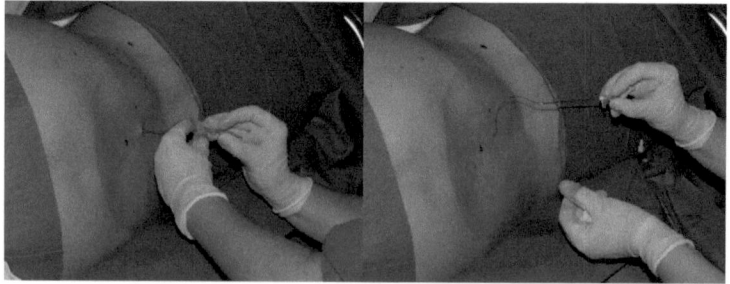

Figure 5. Catheter introduction into the epidural area

After completing the procedure (Figure 6) childbearing woman was laid on her back, and during that time blood pressure, pulse and general condition of the childbearing woman as well as condition of the fetus were monitoring using cardiotocography (CTG). Once the anesthesiologist was assured that the state of childbearing woman and fetus are proper and the epidural block functions orderly, a bolus dose of 8-10 mL of 0.125% solution of *Chirocaine* or *Bupivacaine* was injected. Childbearing woman then had to lie on her back over 10 minutes with a lifted headboard while a sure sign of anestetics having effect was a warm sensation in her legs.

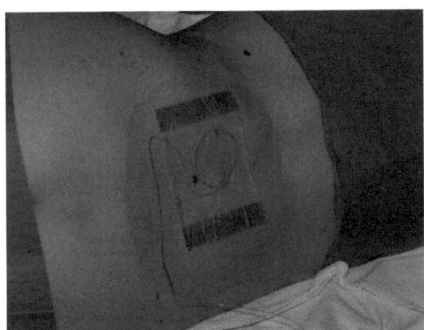

Figure 6. Fixed outer part of epidural catheter

The childbearing women have expressed painfulness of upcoming uterine contractions and efficiency of analgesia through the numerical scale from 0 to 10 according to the visual analogue scale - VAS (93). Finally, the childbearing woman depending on obstetric findings adjusted herself in one of the side positions and was connected to the system for a continuous epidural analgesia. All relevant information related to delivery under an epidural analgesia was registered in a specially designed *Anaesthesiology form* (Figure 7).

Protocol number:	Date:		Anaesthesiologist:	
Medical history registration number:			PIN:	
Name and surname:			Age:	
Profession:	Height [cm]:		Weight [kg]:	
Gestational age [weeks]:	Presentation: 1. Cephalic 2. Breech		Cervical dilation [cm]:	
Number of deliveries:	Previous analgesia: 1. No 2. Satisfactory 3. Unsatisfactory			
Psychophysical preparation: 1. No 2. Antenatal classes 3. In the delivery room				
Indication for EPA: 1. Woman's request 2. Dystocia 3. Other				
Position: 1. Lying 2. Sitting	Interspinous area:	Needle type:		Catheter type:
Analgesic:		Technical difficulties: 1. No 2. Yes (description:)		

Time				
Dose [mL/h]				
Dilation [cm]				
Blood pressure				
Pulse [bpm]				
Analgesia (VAS)				
Mot. blockade				
Temperature				
Shivering				
Nausea				
Somnolence				
Other				
Drugs				
Liquids				
Lab. exams				

Mode of delivery:	1. Spontaneous vaginal	2. Vacuum extraction	3. Caesarean delivery
Episiotomy: 1. No 2. Yes		Other obstetric interventions:	
Sex: 1. Male 2. Female	Weight [g]:	Length [cm]:	Apgar index (1'/5'):
Cardiopulmonary resuscitation (CPR): 1. Not required 2. Aspiration 3. Sensitive stimulation 4. Ventilation 5. Intubation			

Figure 7. *Anaesthesiology form* for monitoring deliveries under epidural analgesia at the Department of Gynecology and Obstetrics, University Hospital Center Rijeka, Croatia

For the purpose of this study, we divided indications for epidural analgesia in two basic groups: medical indications and indications according to the request of childbearing woman. According to the statement of the American College of Obstetricians and Gynecologists (ACOG) and the American Society of Anesthesiologists (ASA) from 2002 for the application of epidural analgesia, other than medical indications and in the absence of contraindications, sufficient is only the wish or request of the childbearing woman (9).

The medical indications group included pathological conditions in pregnancy (pre-eclampsia and other hypertensive disorders during pregnancy, chronic placental insufficiency, intrauterine growth retardation, gestational diabetes), the childbearing woman diseases (cardiac, pulmonary, neurological, and endocrinological, etc.) and pathological conditions in labour (spastic cervical opening, extremely painful contractions and weak cooperation of childbearing woman in the first and second stage of labour, early rupture of membranes with immature cervical opening, previous caesarean section).

In cases when the childbearing woman requested to receive the epidural analgesia none of the abovementioned medical indications were present, and it was the obstetrician who decided about setting the epidural analgesia on the basis of obstetric findings and assessment of fetal condition. Additional criteria for applying the epidural analgesia in aforementioned cases were the active phase of labour with good contractions and dilation of the cervical opening of 3-5 cm. Epidural analgesia was not applied in presence of some of above mentioned contraindications.

Ethical issues

During the research, basic ethical and bioethical principles were respected (personal integrity, justice, charity, and safety) in accordance with the Nuremberg Code and the revised Declaration of Helsinki. Even the data collection was performed in accordance with ethical and bioethical principles wherein it was emphasized that the results publication in professional and scientific publications will be carried out by maintaining the anonymity.

Statistical analysis

The application programme *Statistica, version 10. (Stat. Soft Inc., Tulsa UK, USA)* was used for collected data analysis and *Excel* for graphic displays. In the primary evaluation of results methods of descriptive statistics were used in order to determine the arithmetic values, standard deviations, medians, range and other statistical parameters.

In the comparative performance analysis, depending on the analyzed variables (dependent or independent), *Student t-test* was applied in those cases where a distribution of results was normal and *Mann Whitney U test* from non-parametric tests where a distribution of results was not normal. To verify the relationship between particular variables the *Pearson* product-moment correlation coefficient was calculated. Since the non-numeric (descriptive) data actually categoried within monitoring group that had a common feature selected, their quantification was expressed in proportion or percentage by which their characteristic was represented in the sample. For the analysis of qualitative, categorical (non numerical) data nonparametric X^2 *test* was used, and *Yates* correction only if necessary. For the analysis of results where three variables qualitative comparison was necessary, the ANOVA test was used. Statistical significance was valued as $p < 0.05$ with a confidence interval of 95%.

CHAPTER IV: RESULTS OF THE STUDY

Results

This research included a total number of 2126 patients. From that number 1083 were included in the study group and 1043 in the control group. Epidemiological characteristics of both childbearing women groups are shown in Table 1. There was no difference in age (U = 563656.0), body weight (U = 550493.0) and body mass index (BMI) (U = 553685.0), while the childbearing woman in the control group were statistically slightly taller than childbearing women in study group (U = 535260.5). Representation of primiparous women in the study group was also significantly taller than in the control group (X^2 = 32.74943). The average gestational age was 39.5 weeks for both groups.

Table 1. Epidemiological characteristics of the study and control group of patients (n=2126)

Epidemiological characterictics	Study group (n=1083)	Control group (n=1043)	p
Age (X ± SD)	29 ± 5.0	29 ± 4.7	0.936
Primiparous (%)	81.4	72.7	<0.001
Height /cm/ (X ± SD)	167.3 ± 6.1	168.2 ± 6.1	0.036
Weight /kg/ (X ± SD)	79.5 ± 11.3	80.1 ± 12.0	0.312
BMI (X ± SD)	28.3 ± 3.7	28.4 ± 3.9	0.679

n - number of cases, X ± SD - arithmetic value ± standard deviation, BMI - body mass index,
p - statistical significance (p <0.05)

Observing the course of pregnancies and the frequency of complications we determined that between the study and control group there was no statistically significant difference in the occurrence of hypertensive disorders ($X^2 = 0.18$), previous caesarean section ($X^2 = 1.58$), macrosomia ($X^2 = 0.12$) and gestational diabetes ($X^2 = 0.83$), while cases of chronic placental insufficiency and fetal growth retardation ($X^2 = 5.60$) were significantly higher in the study group. The results are shown in Table 2.

Table 2. Pregnancy course and complications in the study (n = 1083) and control group (n = 1043)

Pregnancy complications	Study group n (%)	Control group n (%)	p
No	766 (70.7)	815 (78.1)	<0.001
Hypertensive disorders	63 (5.8)	66 (6.3)	0.676
Previous caesarean section	114 (10.5)	92 (8.8)	0.209
Placental insufficiency / IUGR	36 (3.3)	17 (1.6)	0.018
Macrosomia	23 (2.1)	19 (1.8)	0.731
GDM	34 (3.1)	25 (2.4)	0.363

n (%) - number of cases (percentage), IUGR – intrauterine growth retardation, GDM – gestational diabetes, p - statistical significance (p <0.05)

Within the primary objective of this research, a comparison between the study and control group with regard to obstetric characteristics was made: onset of delivery, duration of the first and second stages of labour, intrapartum complications and mode of delivery with a focus on operative deliveries. Results

Table 3. Obstetric characteristics of the study (n = 1083) and control group (n = 1043)

Obstetric characteristics	Study group n (%)	Control group n (%)	p
1st stage of labour /min/	480	300	<0.001
median (range)	(65 – 3900)	(55 – 1980)	
2nd stage of labour /min/	38.5	30	<0.001
median (range)	(10 – 280)	(8 – 160)	
Onset of delivery			
- RVP	379 (35.0)	232 (22.3)	<0.001
- contractions	531 (49.0)	781 (74.9)	<0.001
- induction	173 (16.0)	29 (2.8)	<0.001
Vaginal delivery	866 (80.0)	971 (93.1)	<0.001
Vacuum extraction	47 (4.3)	17 (1.6)	<0.001
Caesarean section	170 (15.7)	55 (5.3)	<0.001
- dystocia	99 (58.2)	32 (58.2)	0.885
- fetal distress	62 (36.5)	16 (29.1)	0.359
- other	9 (5.3)	7 (12.7)	0.128
Pathologic CTG finding	186 (17.2)	45 (4.3)	<0.001
Fetal bradycardia	9 (0.8)	12 (1.3)	0.394
Hypotension	1 (0.1)	0 (0)	0.929
Febris sub partu	47 (4.3)	9 (0.9)	<0.001

n (%) - number of cases (percentage), CTG finding - cardiotocographic finding, RVP – premature rupture of membranes, p - statistical significance (p <0.05) are presented in details in Table 3. Thus, in the study group of deliveries under EPA were significantly higher number of deliveries that began with premature rupture of membranes (X^2 = 41.39) and prostaglandin induction (X^2 = 105.89), but there were significantly fewer deliveries that began with spontaneous contractions (X^2 = 149.97). In the same group the arithmetic value of duration of the first stage of labour was 480 minutes, while of the second stage was 38.5 minutes, which was significantly longer than in the control group (U = 312762.0; U = 462195.5). Pathologic cardiotocographic findings (X^2 = 89.84) and operative deliveries i.e. vacuum extraction (X^2 = 13.6) and caesarean section (X^2 = 58.9) were significantly more frequent in deliveries conducted under EPA in comparison with the control group, while the spontaneous vaginal delivery was significantly more frequent in the control group of childbearing women (X^2 = 78.1). Fetal bradycardia as an indication for an urgent caesarean section was not statistically higher in the study group of childbearing women (X^2 = 0.73), while it was also the case with hypotension (X^2 = 0.01), whereas the higher body temperature $\geq 38^0$C was significantly more frequent from the statistic point of view in the study group of childbearing women (X^2 = 23.71). Although dystocia and fetal distress were the most common indications for caesarean section in both groups, there were no statistically significant differences in the frequency of observed indication between the groups (for dystocia X^2 = 0.02; for fetal distress X^2 = 0.84; for other indications X^2 = 2.32).

In the study group of deliveries conducted under epidural analgesia, the duration of the first and second stages of labour was presented, separately for each of the modes of delivery, and the results are shown in Table 4.

The first and second stage of labour were the shortest in the subgroup of spontaneous vaginal deliveries (H = 34.58812; H = 38.13186) and also statistically significantly different in comparison to both types of operative deliveries.

Table 4. Duration of stages of labour given the modes of deliveries in the study group of deliveries under epidural analgesia (n = 1083)

Mode of delivery	Vaginal	VE	SC	p*
1st stage of labour /min/ median (range)	480 (65 – 3000)	499.8 (150 – 1260)	660 (150 – 3900)	<0.001
2nd stage of labour /min/ median (range)	40 (10 – 280)	72 (14 – 210)	81 (25 – 247)	<0.001

VE - vacuum extraction, SC - caesarean section, p* - the ANOVA test statistical significance (p <0.05)

Within the neonatal outcomes framework the birth weight and sex of newborns, frequency of Apgar score <7 in 5th minute, the pH value of fetal and / or umbilical arterial blood <7.20 and neonatal infection were observed, while all results are shown in Table 5. There were no statistically significant differences between the study and control group for none of the examined variables (for birth weight t = 1.16778; for sex X^2 = 0.228; for Apgar score <7 in 5th minute X^2 = 0.332; for fetal/umbilical blood pH X^2 = 0.527; for neonatal infection X^2 = 1.09).

Puerperal complications were observed on the basis of used analgesics and antibiotics as well as the appearance of fever, headache and urinary retention after delivery. By comparing the two groups it was discovered that fever occurrence (X^2 = 8.22) and administration of antibiotics (X^2 = 16.37) were significantly more frequent in the study compared to the control group of puerperal women. On the other side, there were no statistically significant differences between the groups regarding the use of analgesics (X^2 = 0.01), occurrence of headache (X^2 = 0.46) and urinary retention (X^2 = 1.64). Results are presented in Table 6. Among the causes of fever in the puerperal period were diagnosed one case of urinary tract infection, endometritis, mastitis and respiratory infection, while in 17 cases (80.9%) the cause remained unknown.

Table 5. Neonatal characteristics of the study (n = 1083) and control group (n = 1043)

Neonatal characteristics	Study group n (%)	Control group n (%)	p
Birth weight /grams/			
(X ± SD)	3486 ± 484	3462 ± 471	0.243
Sex			0.632
- MALE	551 (50.9)	541 (51,9)	
- FEMALE	532 (49.1)	502 (48,1)	
API 5' < 7	6 (0.5)	4 (0.4)	0.564
Fetal/umbilical pH < 7.20	41 (3.8)	15 (1.4)	0.468
Neonatal infections	83 (7.7)	67 (6.4)	0.297

n (%) - number of cases (percentage), X ± SD - arithmetic value ± standard deviation, API 5' - Apgar score in 5th minute, p - statistical significance (p <0.05)

In the control group there were three cases of endometritis, one case of urinary tract infection while in one case the cause of the fever was not found. In Table 7 are given results of comparing the two groups of respondents whose deliveries were conducted under epidural analgesia because of medical indications or requests or desires of the childbearing woman for analgesia. The first stage of labour lasted significantly longer from statistic point of view (U = 94426.0) and more often the delivery was terminated by caesarean section (X^2 = 19.82) in group A in comparison to group B. Dystocia, as an indication for caesarean section, was statistically significantly more frequent (X^2 = 10.52) in group A in comparison to group B and acute fetal distress (X^2 = 5.04) in group B in comparison with the group A. There were no significant differences between groups in duration of the second stage of labour (U=122301.0).

Table 6. Complications in the study (n = 1083) and control group (n = 1043) of puerperal women

Puerperal complications	Study group n (%)	Control group n(%)	p
Temperature $\geq 38^0$C	21 (1.9)	5 (0.5)	0.004
Administration of analgetics	50 (4.6)	47 (4.5)	0.986
Administration of antibiotics	282 (26.0)	105 (10.1)	<0.001
Headache	2 (0.2)	0 (0)	0.496
Urinary retention	7 (0.6)	2 (0.2)	0.200

n (%) - number of cases (percentage), p - statistical significance (p <0.05)

Spontaneous vaginal delivery was statistically significantly more frequent (X^2 = 22.42) in group B, while the the frequency of vacuum extraction showed no significant difference (X^2 = 1.07) between these groups. When we speak about the perinatal outcome, there was no statistical difference between groups A and B for any of the examined parameters (for birthweight U = 12.00; for newborns sex X^2 = 0.0485; for Apgar score <7 in 5th minute X^2 = 0.11).

When comparing the group of respondents using the epidural analgesia on request and the control group (Table 8) again there were statistically significant differences in the duration of the first (U = 120604.0) and the second stage of labour (U = 139824.0), but not in the frequency of conducted deliveries completed by vacuum extraction (X^2 = 2.60) and caesarean section (X^2 = 3.53). Of indication between groups for cesarean section dystocia was significantly more frequent (X^2 = 10.46) in the control group of, while the acute fetal distress (X^2 = 4.77) in study group. There were no significant differences between indicators of perinatal outcomes (for birthweight U = 168043.5; for newborns sex $X^2 = 0.03546$; for Apgar score <7 in 5th minute $X^2 = 0.25$).

Table 7. Comparison of two groups of deliveries conducted under epidural analgesia (EPA) considering its indication for placing EPA (group A – medical indication, Group B – on request of the childbearing woman)

Obstetric characteristics	Group A (n=744) n(%)	Group B (n=339) n(%)	p
1st stage of labour /min/ median (range)	540 (90 – 3900)	420 (65 – 1440)	<0.001
2nd stage of labour /min/ median (range)	38 (15 – 240)	40 (10 – 280)	0.445
Vaginal delivery	566 (76.1)	300 (88.5)	<0.001
Vacuum extraction	36 (4.8)	11 (3.3)	0.302
Caesarean section	2 (19.1)	28 (8.3)	<0.001
- dystocia	91 (58.2)	8 (28.6)	<0.001
- fetal distress	46 (36.5)	16 (57.1)	0.025
- other	5 (5.3)	4 (14.3)	0.064
Birth weight /grams/ (X ± SD)	3484 ± 506	3492 ± 434	0.533
Sex			0.826
- MALE	377 (50.7)	174 (51.3)	
- FEMALE	367 (49.3)	165 (48.7)	
API 5' < 7	4 (0.5)	2 (0.6)	0.739

n (%) - number of cases (percentage), X ± SD - arithmetic value ± standard deviation, API – Apgar score, p - statistical significance (p <0.05)

Table 8. Comparing the group of deliveries conducted under epidural analgesia (EPA) on request (n = 339) and control group (n=1043)

Obstetric characteristics	Control group n (%)	EPA on request n (%)	p
1st stage of labour /min/ median (range)	300 (55 – 1980)	420 (65 – 1440)	<0.001
2nd stage of labour /min/ median (range)	30 (8 – 160)	40 (10 – 280)	0.001
Vaginal delivery	971 (93.1)	300 (88.5)	<0.001
Vacuum extraction	17 (1.6)	11 (3.2)	0.107
Caesarean section	55 (5.3)	28 (8.3)	0.063
- dystocia	32 (58.2)	8 (28.6)	0.001
- fetal distress	16 (29.1)	16 (57.1)	0.029
- other	7 (12.7)	4 (14.3)	0.861
Birth weight (g) (X ± SD)	3462 ± 471	3492 ± 434	0.163
Sex			0.851
- MALE	541 (51.9)	174 (51.3)	
- FEMALE	502 (48.1)	165 (487)	
API 5' <7	4 (0.4)	2 (0.6)	0.979

n (%) - number of cases (percentage), X ± SD - arithmetic value ± standard deviation, API – Apgar score, p - statistical significance (p <0.05)

A special group of vaginal deliveries (group C) was formed from the study group of deliveries (n = 1083) in which epidural analgesia was reduced /

discontinuated at the end of the first stage of labour where the cervix was opened by 7-8 cm or during the early phase of the second stage of labour.

By comparing the aforementioned group of deliveries and group of remaining deliveries conducted under epidural analgesia (group D), no statistically significant differences in the frequency of certain modes of deliveries - vaginal delivery ($X^2 = 0.75$), vacuum extraction ($X^2 = 1.01$) and caesarean delivery ($X^2 = 2.59$) were found. The results are shown in Table 9.

Table 9. Comparison of two groups of deliveries under epidural analgesia (EPA) with discontinuation (group C) and without discontinuation the epidural infusion (group D) regarding mode of delivery (n = 1083)

Mode of delivery	Group C (n=225)	Group D (n=858)	p
	n (%)	n (%)	
Vaginal delivery	185 (82.2)	681 (79.4)	0.391
Vacuum extraction	13 (5.8)	34 (4.0)	0.315
Caesarean section	27 (12.0)	143 (16.7)	0.107

n (%) - number of cases (percentage), p - statistical significance (p <0.05)

CHAPTER V: DISCUSSION AND REFERENCES

Discussion

By introducing the epidural analgesia in delivery rooms around the world, more and more authors in their papers reported about its favorable effects on the course and outcome of labour, which resulted in conclusion about epidural analgesia as one of the most effective method of birth pain control (12, 26, 86,

90, 94). Thus, many reports show a significant increase in a share of deliveries that were in any way connected with continuous epidural analgesia (42, 67, 72, 73, 95). Nulliparity and local cultural heritage were marked as important factors affecting the prevalence of its use (85). Various changes in obstetric approach, regional analgesia techniques and the beginning of their implementation in order to eliminate pain in delivery as well as administered medicines were introduced with the aim of obtaining greater efficiency, better tolerability and lesser common side effects (19, 66, 78, 87, 88, 89, 96-98, 99). It seems that an optimal solution for the problem of birth pain was found, and which could stop or at least slow the trend of rising frequency of operative interventions during deliveries, especially caesarean sections, and also reduce intrapartum and postpartum administration of analgesics and antibiotics (98).

Considering the purpose of introduction the epidural analgesia was to reduce the frequency of specific medical interventions during deliveries, we remained surprised with somehow contradictory reports of several authors that highlighted the fact that the frequency of operative deliveries had not decreased, but started to increase (66, 83, 88, 90, 100, 101). Differences in the results and conclusions of some authors should be sought at diverse plans and methodologies of studies, number of respondents, the chosen control groups, and the individual's choices to promote a method or to try to diminish its value. The important impact could also be clinical attitudes and doctrines which the individual authors follow in their obstetric work, particularly with regard to assessment of indications for operative deliveries (78, 98, 102). The frequency of caesarean section and vacuum extraction and their mutual relationship will depend on the fact how much the vacuum extraction is or is not "popular" or ignored in some obstetric practicing institutions. The available diagnostic fetal distress and vulnerability evaluation methods can undoubtedly influence the results of clinical research on the need for operative termination of delivery conducted under epidural analgesia. Those obstetricians who base their decisions to operatively terminate deliveries exclusively on clinical indicators of fetal compromise (meconium amniotic fluid, abnormal fetal heart rates controlled with obstetric headphones or using cardiotocography) and who do not use vacuum extraction, specify higher frequency of caesarean section than those who use determination of fetal blood acid-base status to assess fetal risk and to whom the vacuum extraction is a normal and safe way to end delivery with appropriate strict indications.

Continuous epidural analgesia was introduced at our Department as a routine in obstetrics at the end of 2001. Its systematic and continuous administration enabled us to gain our own experiences with the aforementioned method of the birth pain control.

After the 10-year period, we decided to start a study on the basis of carefully prepared and detailed medical records data on vaginal deliveries conducted under continuous epidural analgesia. The basic aim of this study was to objectively evaluate the need for surgically completion of the delivery conducted under the epidural analgesia, and to determine their frequency. Then, we investigated how much the classical principles and criteria of conducting the vaginal delivery can be responsible for obstetric operations in the final stage of such deliveries, due to which we tested the hypothetical connection between the increased frequency of operative interventions and classical conduction of delivery under the epidural analgesia. For such a scientific and research project adequate conditions were needed and should have been created. We consider our advantage in comparison to other studies in fact that our institution has low incidence of caesarean section (from 10-12%) which in our opinion guarantees that all obstetric interventions were strictly medically indicated and justified. Another favorable fact of this study is that the frequency of vacuum extraction in our institution is maintained for years at the level of ≤2%. Adequately large sample of childbearing women (more than 2000) was included in this research. After a detailed explanation about the effect of epidural analgesia and

38

introducing the epidural catheter all the childbearing women in study group have signed the consent for the aforementioned invasive procedure, and that should be a standard practice in all delivery rooms (97, 103). The control group was harmonized with the study groups regarding the age of childbearing women and their constitutional characteristics in order to eliminate or substantially reduce their potential impact on the course and outcome of labour. The study and control groups of childbearing women were equalized in comparison to their age (29 years in average), body weight and body mass index, while the participants were on average only 1cm lower in comparison with the childbearing women from the control group. Due to the fact that the different duration of pregnancy could affect the results, both groups were harmonized in regard to the average gestational age that corresponded to the foreseen pregnancy, which was also a frequent criterion in other studies (40, 68, 78, 90, 91, 98, 99, 102). In order to homogenize the study groups additionally, we were performing strict inclusion criteria: singleton pregnancy at ≥35 gestational weeks and a healthy fetus at cephalic position. We tried to balance the study group and the control group regarding pregnancies with complications and analysed separately stated gestational disorders and their consequences which can change the course and outcome of the labour. However, some studies state that there is a possibility that maternal and fetal factors are more responsible for the higher rate of caesarean section than the epidural analgesia itself (94, 100). In both examined groups of pregnancies similar frequencies of hypertensive disorders, gestational diabetes, macrosomia and deliveries after previous caesarean sections were all without statistical significance. The only complication in pregnancy with a significantly higher frequency of occurrences in the study group was a chronic placental insufficiency with fetal growth retardation, because we consider it one of indications from the list of medical indications for use of continuous epidural analgesia in induced delivery. However, due to the fact that each of the observed complications of pregnancies in the study group had a somewhat higher frequency, their cumulative percentage shows a higher frequency in total, in comparison with the control group, where is subsequently recorded a significantly higher proportion of pregnancies with normal clinical course and outcome.

The most important results of this study, and the primary objective, was obtained by comparing deliveries under continuous epidural analgesia and control group of deliveries in term of duration of the first and second stages of labour, intrapartum complications and operative deliveries. By calculating median values we have shown that the first stage of labour lasted significantly longer (480 min) from statistic point of view in the study than in the control group. Also the second stage of labour had a significantly longer duration and lasted 38.5 min. There is a possibility that activity of continuous epidural analgesia has reduced the intensity of contractions thus prolonged the first stage of labour in comparison to the control group where the median value of the first stage of labour duration was shorter for 3 hours. A significantly higher prevalence of primiparous women, deliveries which started with a spontaneous rupture of membranes and leakage of amniotic fluid as well as deliveries induced with prostaglandins could have influence on the prolonged duration of the first stage of labour (98, 104). The uncertainties regarding criteria for determining the onset of delivery (98) should be emphasized, which in our study are strictly defined as regular contractions at intervals of 10 min. However, the trend of prolonged duration of delivery following the epidural analgesia even without mentioned obstetric factors and their potential impact can also be seen in papers of other authors (21).

When we speak about the second stage of labour that is significantly longer in the study group in comparison with the control group, should be said that the regional anesthesia had a crucial influence on the slow progress of delivery from the beginning of the second stage of labour. Zhang et al. arrived to equal conclusion by examining duration and mode of delivery in two groups of primiparous women with singleton pregnancy and fetal head in forward position, with or without the epidural analgesia (38). The negative impact of epidural analgesia on the second stage of labour is even more probable if we remember that in our study group there was neither greater incidence of gestational diabetes, macrosomia or nor delivery upon the previous caesarean section (105). Almost the same average birth weight in both groups is a clear confirmation that fetal weight was not a factor which influenced on duration and frequency of operative deliveries. It is well known that, besides it reduces birth pain, continuous epidural analgesia block motor fibres of sacral nerves during the first stage of labour so in case of accelerated absorption of local anesthetics in the epidural space its effect can be cumulative and persist through the second stage of labour. So the sense and reflex neuromuscular mechanisms that under physiological conditions increase the uterine expulsion force by activating the muscles of the childbearing woman abdominal wall can weaken (18). Suppression of above described very important physiological reflexes in the final stage of labour and disruption of coordination between uterine contractions, instinctive and wilful pushing by childbearing woman, a continuous epidural analgesia may delay or stop the process of delivery that under normal conditions is a self-limiting act of nature (97). It is not surprising that the results of our research pointed to the real problem of significantly increased operative interventions in the final stages of vaginal deliveries under the epidural analgesia. So both vacuum extraction with 4.3% and caesarean section with 15.7% were three times more frequent in the study in comparison with the control group. Even other authors reported about the similar results (90, 98). About the reliability of our results related to the clinical justification for caesarean section, testifies a low overall annual frequency of caesarean section which in 2009 and 2010 was 12.9% and 11.7%, respectively. However, when analyzing the most common indications for caesarean section, then dystocia and fetal distress were slightly more frequent in the study group but have not reached the statistical difference with respect to the control group. It can thus be concluded that continuous epidural analgesia has not significantly increased the participation of dystocia and fetal distress among the indications for an emergency caesarean section. Accordingly, other indications were more frequent in the control group but also with no statistical significance. Contrary to the aforementioned results are data on significantly higher frequency of pathologic cardiotocographic records in deliveries that were conducted under the continuous epidural analgesia, but everything is clearer when it is known that routinely such records were verified with intrapartum applied scalp pH-metric method and determining the acid-base state of the fetus. In fact, by comparing two groups of deliveries and within the presented neonatal outcome we have shown that there were no statistically significant differences in the percentage of fetal acidosis which is consistent with data from the literature (98). Likewise, it should be noted that there were neither significant differences in the occurrence of fetal bradycardia that will be the reason to undertake an urgent caesarean section. This is also a confirmation that unnecessary obstetric interventions can be avoided by a use of the fetal scalp pH metric method in the interest of the mother and fetus. Hypotension at childbearing woman after introducing a continuous epidural analgesia was extremely rare and has not represented a greater practical problem, probably because of high quality preparation and preliminary actions undertaken to prevent the aforementioned complications. On the other side, fever at childbearing woman whose frequency was 4.5 times higher than in the control group may be considered a specific complication of epidural analgesia (40, 41). The obtained result goes in favor of the opinion of many that the fever at childbearing woman delivering under epidural analgesia is usually not caused by an infection, but is a direct result of activity of administered drug which causes a dysfunction of the thermoregulatory center (98).

After the first and the second stage of labour being analyzed separately for every mode of delivery, the shortest duration was measured in the group of spontaneous vaginal deliveries (480 min and 40 min, respectively), while statistically longer were both stages in group where deliveries were finished by vacuum extraction (about 500 min and 72 min, respectively) and caesarean section (660 min and 81 min, respectively). It could be concluded that the duration of the first and particularly the second stage of labour was almost twice as long in the groups of operative deliveries, and made an adverse effect on the mode of delivery, if we consider that the vacuum extraction and caesarean section are particularly undesirable "outcome". In other words, it seems that a significant extension of particularly the second stage of labour considerably reduces chances for a spontaneous vaginal delivery, and increases chances for obstetric intervention (80).

Due to unquestionable specific needs for a continuous epidural analgesia in deliveries in which there is a medical indication for its use we wanted to investigate how much the existence of some of the medical indications affects the course of such deliveries, duration of labour stages and the mode of deliveries. Among the most common indications were stronger birth pain due to spastic cervical opening with the cervical dilation of 3-5 cm, immature cervix at induced deliveries and scars following the previous caesarean sections, of gestational disorders we can speak about hypertensive conditions, gestational diabetes and fetal growth retardation, whilst when speaking about mothers' diseases, various orthopedic and ophthalmic diagnosis, as well as neurological, pulmonary, and cardiac diseases which due to a strong sympathetic stimulation could enter in a phase of decompensation. For this purpose we have divided deliveries under epidural analgesia to those with medical indication and those without medical indication where the regional analgesia was administered only on the request of the childbearing woman. In the following text, we compared a group of deliveries under epidural analgesia given on childbearing woman request with a group of deliveries in which we applied analgesia for medical reasons and the control group regarding their obstetric characteristics. The results showed that in the group of deliveries under continuous epidural analgesia which was given according to the childbearing woman wish the duration of the first labour stage was significantly shorter; the rate of spontaneous vaginal deliveries was higher, while the rate of caesarean section was more than twice lower in comparison to group of deliveries under epidural analgesia given for medical indications. The differences itself were statistically significant. Dystocia was statistically higher in the group with medical indication for administration of epidural analgesia, while acute fetal distress and other indications for caesarean section were more frequent in the group under epidural analgesia given according to childbearing woman request. We explain the aforementioned results with a high proportion of spastic/rigid cervix as a specific indication among medical indications for a continuous epidural analgesia, as indirectly indicated a significantly longer duration of the first stage of labour in the same group of deliveries (106-109).

By comparing the same group of deliveries under epidural analgesia given on childbearing woman request with the control group of deliveries without epidural analgesia, we avoided all conditions i.e. all medical indications for administering epidural analgesia that could adversely affect the examined obstetric indicators, while eventual presence of disorders of pregnancy is reduced to a minimum. In such conditions, we found that duration of both labour stages lasted statistically longer, that the incidence of spontaneous vaginal deliveries was significantly lower, and that the frequency of caesarean section was significantly higher and at the margin of statistical significance in the group of deliveries that received continuous epidural analgesia. We consider the obtained results probably the best confirmation of an important influence of continuous epidural analgesia regarding the extension of the first and second stages of labour and completion of delivery by caesarean section, which can not be stated for the use of vacuum extraction. Decision to use vacuum extraction is a very specific clinical decision, so the incidence of such procedures among ways of completing deliveries is relative and often difficult to compare. Namely, in those institutions where physicians respect strict indications for using vacuum extraction, and where a good practical training is present, frequency of caesarean section will be definitely lower, while in those centers that slightly neglect the use of vacuum extraction, the only solution for a safe and rapid termination of delivery will be the caesarean section so then its rate/incidence will be higher. Physicians, who relatively liberally use the vacuum extraction even in obstetric circumstances that are not considered as a "real" indication, will have the higher rate of vacuum extraction. For example, Liu et al. described greater number of operative vaginal deliveries under epidural analgesia in nulliparous women, although they did not state what the general incidence of vacuum extractions in their institute really is (60). At our Department, we do not use vacuum extraction too liberally, but we give it an advantage over the caesarean section, whenever there are appropriate obstetric conditions present. Therefore we consider our results regarding the frequency of the vacuum extraction in deliveries with and without continuous epidural analgesia as reliable ones. Thus we are not surprised by literary reports about different experiences related to the influence of epidural analgesia to the caesarean section i.e. a way of completing delivery using instrumental modes of termination (60, 83, 86, 88, 90, 98, 100, 101, 110, 111).

In order to reduce a number of unnecessary obstetric interventions, there is a need of considering possible preventive measures against prolonging the labour stages, particularly the second one as well as eventual change of the classical obstetric attitude and approach in conducting vaginal deliveries.

In order to prevent a prolonged duration of the labour stages, and providing that we keep on the basic reasons for the use of continuous epidural analgesia i.e. removing the birth pain and ending the "vicious circle", then it would be understandable to use an epidural analgesia until it performs its main function and accelerates the progress of labour in its active phase of painful cervical opening. Likewise, a logical question arises about the discontinuation of continuous epidural analgesia at the moment the consistency of cervical tissue changes or when the cervix is sufficiently opened, which is usually considered to be a dilation of 7-8 cm. The idea is, to recover neuroendogenous reflex which due to distension of the vaginal walls increases the secretion of oxytocin from the neurohypophyseos thus intensifying the efficiency of contractions, and to stop inhibition of the previously described reflex mechanism responsible for activation of the abdominal muscles which increases the muscular power of fetus expulsion for 3-4 times in relation to the force of uterine contractions themselves. Such active approach could shorten the first stage of labour, thus entering the second stage of labour with more efficient forces for fetal expulsion. Theoretically, good contractions in the second stage of labour with the absence of cephalopelvic disproportion, deflection or malrotation of the fetal head should be a guarantee of limited duration of the second stage of labour and reduced number of operative interventions that will then remain reserved only for accidental cases of acute fetal endangerment (102, 112-114). Reflections on the discontinuation of continuous epidural analgesia near the end of the first stage of delivery (when cervical dilation is 8 cm) or at the beginning of the second stage of labour are not rare in the literature. The idea is based on a logical assumption that by interrupting the epidural infusion is enabling a faster recovery of the previously inactivated reflex mechanisms that are necessary for the active engagement of childbearing woman in the final stage of delivery. The final opinions on the effectiveness of such procedure are still considered not unanimous but contradictory (11, 39, 98).

Wishing to verify by ourselves any possible and beneficial effects of stopping the epidural infusion of anesthetics on the course of the second stage of labour and delivery outcomes, we divided the study group of vaginal deliveries to those in which the childbearing women received continuous epidural analgesia until the end of delivery and those where childbearing women were not given the continuous epidural analgesia after dilation of cervical opening was determined to be 7-8(10) cm, thus comparing them with regard to obstetric interventions in the final stage of delivery. Although the frequency of caesarean section was higher in the subgroup of deliveries that was conducted to the very end under the epidural analgesia, and the frequency of vacuum extraction was greater in the subgroup of delivery without the continuous epidural analgesia in the second stage of labour, there were no statistically significant differences among them. This suggests that discontinuation of the continuous epidural analgesia at the end of the first stage of labour or at the beginning of the second stage of labour as a universal recommendation chances for caesarean delivery may be reduced, but not significantly affect the overall incidences of operative deliveries, which were 17.8% and 20.6%, respectively (Table 9). According to the results of our research seems that duration of the second stage of labour that is longer than 70-80 min increases the chances of operative deliveries, but it does not mean that after that time, with favourable conditions and correction of certain obstetric factors, one can not expect a spontaneous vaginal delivery. Therefore, a second preventive measure that seems reasonable is a professional recommendation that there is no need to keep strictly a classical attitude about the longest 2-hour duration of the second stage of labour when delivery is conducted under a continuous epidural analgesia, but clinical decisions on process and monitoring of such deliveries should be individualized depending on the present obstetric factors. Thus the epidural analgesia can be continued even in the second stage of labour at regular, efficient and oxytocin stimulated contractions and continuous progression of delivery. In the absence of signs of acute fetal distress, delivery can be waited even after 70-80 min of the end of the second stage of labour. There are good clinical experiences with verticalization of the childbearing women during the final stage of labouring (97). However, in cases of prolonged first stage of labour, relative weakness of uterine contractions despite long-term oxytocin stimulation, malposition of the fetal head and a slow progression of the second stage of labour, we advise clinical caution and closing the epidural infusion of anesthetics in order to increase the success rate of vaginal deliveries i.e. to reduce invasive medical interventions. Active approach is also suggested by other authors (39, 42, 97, 115-117). The proposed individualisation of clinical decisions and procedures when using the continuous epidural analgesia in vaginal deliveries seems to us important and real because it takes into account the existence of differences between childbearing women and their deliveries in terms of epidemiological characteristics but also from the obstetric aspects. It should be taken into account the possibility of different responses to common concentrations and doses epiduraly administered anesthetics but also possible errors in dosing and timing of anesthetics administration (47, 88, 118).

Besides impacts on the course and mode of delivery, when we speak about continuous epidural analgesia, it is necessary to evaluate its safety profile, since it is an invasive procedure with its own contraindications (refusing by childbearing woman, hypovolemia after bleeding, coagulation disorders and anticoagulant therapy, local infection, some neurological and neuromuscular diseases such as multiple sclerosis, tumors, etc.), but also specific complications, such as hypotension, itching, vomiting, toxic reactions, dural puncture and cerebrospinal fluid outflow, total spinal block, epidural hemorrhage, infection (4, 97, 119).

We have examined the safety of epidural analgesia in obstetrics by analysing the neonatal outcome and puerperal complications. Analysing neonatal outcome, we compared the birth weight, gender, Apgar score <7 in 5th minute, pH values of fetal/umbilical cord blood as well as the presence of neonatal infection and found that between the study and control groups there were no statistically significant differences. Many other authors reported identical experiences (21, 113).

Puerperal complications were observed due to the occurrence of fever, headache, urinary retention and use of antibiotics and analgesics. According to obtained results, headache and urinary retention were not more common in the puerperal study group and there was even no need for a more frequent administration of analgesics compared to the control group. Although epidural analgesia and instrumental deliveries are identified as independent risk factors for a post puncture headache and urinary retention, the results can be explained by a high expertise and skills of anesthesiologists as well as with effective preventive measures (32, 35-37). In the contrary, the febrile state and administering antibiotics during the peripartal period of study group were significantly more likely than those in the control group. Such a result could have been expected and can be explained by the significantly higher occurrence of fever during delivery in these groups of childbearing women, whilst increased use of antibiotics in puerperium seems as its direct consequence. A high percentage of postpartum fever of unexplained cause in the study group ($>80\%$) is more a proof in favour of a specific relationship between fever and use of continuous epidural analgesia at childbearing women, but it does not excuses, we can freely say, a broad and liberal use of antibiotics (40, 41).

In the light of presented results, it can be argued that continuous epidural analgesia although invasive procedure is safe enough when applied in delivery. Due to its proven high efficiency, it should be considered as the first method of choice for a reliable delivery analgesia, and this is stated as a common conclusion in the professional literature (3, 4, 82, 86). The neonatal outcome also confirms that continuous epidural analgesia has no adverse effects on neonatal outcome if used under adequate circumstances. Studies of other authors also proved those results (13, 14, 58, 78, 113).

Summarizing the complete results of this study, and taking into account the limitations in terms of a larger number of primiparous women and a smaller number of deliveries initiated by spontaneous contractions in the study group, and the fact that it is not a randomized controlled study (which may hardly acceptable from the ethical point of view or even unacceptable, because the needed/desired epidural analgesia shall be rejected for some childbearing women), we found that the use of continuous epidural analgesia in deliveries can significantly prolong the first and second stage of labour and increase the rate of operative deliveries, particularly caesarean section. However, there was a doubt, as was the case in many previous studies, that the described results may have been influenced by the fact of a higher percentage of certain pathologic conditions of pregnancy and delivery (hypertensive disorders, previous caesarean delivery, gestational diabetes, macrosomia, fetal growth retardation, spastic/rigid cervix). So we planned and designed this clinical and scientific study with proper and genuine selection of study and control groups of childbearing women and their deliveries, being able to prove that continuous epidural analgesia with clear and beneficial effects in terms of labour analgesia has an undoubtedly important and almost decisive influence on prolongation of the first and second stages of labour and increased frequency of deliveries completed by caesarean section.

By analyzing the results, we confirmed the hypothesis from the beginning of the research about an uncritical use of epidural analgesia and a "blind" application of the criteria of classical obstetrics for expectant conduction of such vaginal deliveries as a crucial factor of adverse effects on duration of delivery and frequency of operative interventions. In conclusion, we would like to emphasize that instead of non-selective and completely uniform application of continuous epidural analgesia in vaginal deliveries, every parturient woman, depending on specificities of her obstetric situations, has to be approached individually in order to reduce its negative, unwanted and side effects. With such committed professional approach we will be able to make a step further in efforts to advance the process of humanization in obstetrics that much needed in this sphere of human activities.

Conclusion

Continuous epidural analgesia administered in vaginal deliveries has significantly prolonged duration of the first and second stage of labour in comparison with the control group. The result was identical even after comparison with the control group of deliveries in which epidural analgesia was administered only because of the request of childbearing woman. The incidence of operative obstetric interventions in the final stage of delivery in terms of an emergency caesarean section and instrumental vaginal delivery has increased significantly (3 times) with the use of continuous epidural analgesia. Among indications for caesarean section, dystocia and acute fetal distress were the most frequent indications in the group of deliveries conducted under epidural analgesia. By comparing the two groups of deliveries under continuous epidural analgesia due to medical indications i.e. on the request of the childbearing woman, in the first group dystocia was statistically significantly higher, whilst in the second group of deliveries it was acute fetal distress. The results showed that a significant extension of the second stage of labour (>70-80 min) increases the chances of operative deliveries, especially if continuous epidural analgesia is applied uncritically and if is insisting on a strict enforcement of the classic criteria for conducting the vaginal delivery regarding duration of the second stage of labour.

Among the observed intrapartum complications, only the fever of $\geq 38^0 \mathrm{C}$ as apparently specific complication of epidural analgesia was significantly higher in the study group compared to the control group of childbearing women.

There were no statistically significant differences between the study and the control group regarding the neonatal outcomes, so it can be concluded that from the aforementioned neonatal aspect, the continuous epidural analgesia is a safe method of delivery pain control.

Among postpartum complications, only the fever and subsequent use of antibiotics were much more present after delivery conducted under continuous epidural analgesia.

Based on the results of this research we recommend an active and individualized approach that respects diversities and specificities of each childbearing woman as well as particular obstetric situations, with the aim of shortening the first and especially the second stage of labour and reduce the application of emergency obstetric interventions in the final stage of vaginal deliveries.

References

1. Doughty A. Walter Stoeckel (1871–1961): A pioneer of regional analgesia in obstetrics. Anaesthesia 1990;45:468-71.

2. Curelaru I, Sandu L. Eugen Bogdan Aburel (1899–1975). The pioneer of regional analgesia for pain relief in childbirth. Anaesthesia 1982;37:663-9.

3. Collis R, Plaat F, Urquhart J. Textbook of Obstetric Anesthesia. London: Greenwich Medical Media Ltd 2002;57-70.

4. Wagih M. Obstetric regional anesthesia. ASJOG 2005;(2):8-12.

5. Yantis S, Hirsch N, Smith G. Anesthesia and Intensive Care. 3rd Edition, London Elsevier Ltd 2004.

6. Gonar C, Fernandez C. Epidural analgesia-anesthesia in obstetrics. Eur J Anesthesiol 2000;17:542-58.

7. Matanić-Manestar M, Begović-Sišul E. Epiduralna analgezija u porođaju. Gynaecol Perinatol 2003;12(1);166.

8. Matanić-Manestar M, Begović-Sišul E, Sindik N. Porodna analgezija. Gynaecol Perinatol 2006;15(1):48-51.

9. ACOG practice bulletin Obstetrics analgesis and anesthesia. Int J Gynecol Obstet 2002;78:321-5.

10. Horowitz RH, Yoger Y, Ben–Haroush A, Kaplan B. Women's altitude toward analgesis during labour – a comparison between 1995 and 2001. Eur Obstet Gynaecol 2004;117:30-2.

11. Alexander JM, Sharma SK, McIntire DD, Leveno KJ. Epidural analgesia lenghthens the Friedman active phase of labor. Obstet Gynecol 2002;100:46-50.

12. Anim-Somuah M, Smyth R, Howel C. Epidural versus non-epidural or no analgesia in labour. Cochrane Database Syst Rev 2005;19:CD000331.

13. Cambic CR, Wong CA. Labour analgesia and obstetric outcomes. Br J Anaesth 2010;105(1):50-60.

14. Reynolds F. Labour analgesia and the baby: good news is no news. J Obstet Anesth 2011;20(1):38-50.

15. Meuser T, Wiese R, Molitor D, Ground S, Stamer UM. A survey of labour pain management in Germany. Schmerz 2008;22:184-90.

16. American College of Obstetricians and Gynecologists. Pain relief during labor. ACOG Commitee Opinion 231. Obstet Gynecol 2004;104:213.

17. Cohain JS. The epidural trip: why are so many women taking dangerous drugs during labor? Midwifery Today Int Midwife 2010;(95):21-4.

18. Ranasinghe JS, Birnbach DJ. Progress in analgesia for labor: focus on neuraxial blocks. Int J Womens Health 2010;1:31-43.

19. Gojnic M, Mostic T, Arsenijevic S, Pervulov M, Petković S, Ivanisevic M. Epidural anesthesia from an obstetrics point of view. Clin Exp Obstet Gynecol 2005;32:126-8.

20. Wong CA. Advances in labor analgesia. Int J Womens Health 2010;1:139-54.

21. Gizzo S, Di Gangi S, Saccardi C, Patrelli TS, Paccagnella G, Sansone L et al. Epidural analgesia during labour: Impact on delivery outcome, neonatal well-being, and early breastfeed. Breastfeed Med 2011;13(Epub ahead of print).

22. Caliskan E, Ozdamar D, Doger E, Cakiroglu Y, Kus A, Corakci A. Prospective case control comparison of fetal intrapartum oxygen saturations during epidural analgesia. Int J Obstet Anesth 2010;19(1):77-81.

23. Lim Y, Chakravarty S, Ocampo CE, Sia AT. Comparison of automated intermittent low volume bolus with continuous infusion for labour epidural analgesia. Anaesth Intensive Care 2010;38(5):894-9.

24. Capogna G, Camorcia M, Stirparo S, Farcomeni A. Programmed intermittent epidural bolus versus continuous epidural infusion for labor analgesia: the effects on maternal motor function and labor outcome. A randomized double-blind study in nulliparous women. Anesth Analg 2011;113(4):826-31.

25. Rees SG, Collis RE, Spinal cord injury after accidental dural puncture for labor analgesia. Int J Obstet Anesth 2007;16(2):193-5.

26. Leo S, Sia AT. Maintaining labour epidural analgesia: what is the best opinion? Curr Opin Anesthesiol 2008;21(3):263-9.

27. Skrablin S, Grgic O, Mihaljevic S, Blajic J. Comparison of intermittent and continuous epidural analgesia on delivery and progression of labour. J Obstet Gynaecol 2011;31(2):134-8.

28. Franchi F, Ibrahim B, Rossi F, Maspero ML, Morabito O, Asti D et al. Coagulation testing before epidural analgesia at delivery: cost analysis. Thromb Res 2011;128(1):18-20.

29. Vincent RD, Chestnut DH. Epidural analgesia and labor. Am Fam Physic 1998;58:1785-92.

30. Jorda Sanz L, Gallego Garcia J, Leon Crasi I, Abengochea Cotaina A. Blood patch in a patient with postdural puncture headache. Rev Esp Anesthesiol Reanim 2006;53(10):678-9.

31. Valldeperas MI, Aguilar JL. Postdural puncture headache in obstetrics: is it really a "benign" complication, and how can we prevent and treat it effectively? Rev Esp Anesthesiol Reanim 2006;53(10):615-7.

32. Van de Velde M, Schepers R, Berends N, Vandermeersch E, De Buck F. Ten years of experience with accidental dural puncture and post-dural puncture headache in a tertiary obstetric anaesthesia department. Int J Obstet Anesth 2008;17(4):329–35.

33. Weil L, Gracer RI, Frauwirth N. Transforaminal epidural blood patch. Pain Physician 2007;10(4):579-82.

34. Chen LK, Huang CH, Jean WH, Lu CW, Lin CJ, Sun WZ. Effective epidural blood patchvolumes for postdural puncture headache in Taiwanese women. J Formos Med Assoc 2007;106(2):134-40.

35. Charlier V, Brichant G, Dewandre PY, Foidart JM, Brichant JF. Obstetrical epidural analgesia and postpartum backache. Rev Med Liege 2012;67(1):16-20.

36. Carley ME, Carley JM, Vasdev G, Lesnick TG, Webb MJ, Ramin KD et al. Factors that are associated with clinically overt postpartum urinary retention after vaginal delivery. Am J Obstet Gynecol 2002;187(2):430-3.

37. Yip SK, Sahota D, Chang A, Chung T. Four-year folow-up of women who were diagnosed to have postpatrum urinary retention. Am J Obstet Gynecol 2002;187(3):648-52.

38. Zhang J, Yancey MK, Klebenoff MA, Schwarz J, Schweitzer D. Does epidural analgesia prolong labor and increase risk of cesarean delivery? A natural experiment. Am J Obstet Gynecol 2001;185:128-34.

39. Plunkett BA, Lin A, Wong CA, Grobman WA, Peaceman AM, Management of the second stage of labour in nulliparas with continuous epidural analgesia. Obstet Gynecol 2003;120:109-14.

40. Riley LE, Celi AC, Onderdonk AB, Roberts DJ, Johnson LC, Tsen LC et al. Association of epidural-related fever and noninfectious inflammation in term labor. Obstet Gynecol 2011;117(3):588-95.

41. Wang LZ, Hu XX, Liu X, Qian P, Ge JM, Tang BL. Influence of epidural dexamethasone on maternal temperature and serum cytokine concentration after labor epidural analgesia. Int J Gynecol Obstet 2011;113(1):40-3.

42. Impely L, MacQuillan K, Robson M. Epidural analgesia need not increase operative delivery rates. Am J Obstet Gynecol 2000;182:358-63.

43. Simmons SW, Cyna AM, Dennis AT, Hughes D. Combined spinal-epidural versus analgesia in labour. Cochrane Database Syst Rev 2003;(4):CD003401.

44. Lewis M, Calthorpe N. Combined spinal epidural analgesia in labour. Fetal Maternal Med Rev 2005;16(1):29-50.

45. Kuyumcuoglu C, Gurbet A, Turker G, Sahin S. The relationship of combined spinal-epidural analgesia and low-back pain after vaginal delivery. Agri 2006;18(3):24-9.

46. Aust H, Plöger B, Frietsch T. Epidural anesthesia in obststrics: an accidentally placed intrathecal catheter – remove it or use it? Z Geburtsh Neonatol 2010;214:249-51.

47. Van den Berg AA, Ghatge S, Armendariz G, Cornelius D, Wang S. Responses to dural puncture during institution of combined spinal-epidural analgesia: a comparison of 27 gauge pencil-point and 27 gauge cutting-edge needles. Anaesth Intensive Care 2011;39(2):247-51.

48. Russell IF. A prospective controlled study of continuous spinal analgesia versus repeat epidural analgesia after accidental dural puncture in labour. Int J Obstet Anesth 2012;21(1):7-16.

49. Kuczkowski KM, Fernández CL. Precipitous delivery after induction of combined spinal-epidural analgesia. Arch Gynecol Obstet 2011;283(2):401.

50. Van de Velde M. Combined spinal-epidural analgesia for labor and delivery: balanced view based on experience and literature. Acta Anaesthesiol Belg 2009;60(2):109-22.

51. Vernon HR, Peter HP, Medge DO, Melvin HS, Lynne H, Britany C. Neostigmine decreases bupivacain use by patient-controlled epidural analgesia during labour: Randomised controlled study. Anesth Analg 2009;109(2):524-31.

52. Haydon ML, Larson D, Reed E, Shrivastava VK, Preslicka CW, Nageotte MP. Obstetric outcomes and maternal satisfaction in nulliparous women using patient-controlled epidural analgesia. Am J Obstet Gynecol 2011;205(3):271-6.

53. Brogly N, Schiraldi R, Vazquez B, Perez J, Guasch E, Gilsanz F. A randomized control trial of patient-controlled epidural analgesia (PCEA) with and without a background infusion using levobupivacaine and fentanyl. Minerva Anestesiol 2011;77(12):1149-54.

54. Leo S, Ocampo CE, Lim Y, Sia AT. A randomized comparison of automated intermittent mandatory boluses with a basal infusion in combination with patient-controlled epidural analgesia for labor and delivery. Int J Obstet Anesth 2010; 19(4):357-64.

55. Srivastava U, Gupta A, Saxena S, Kumar A, Singh S, Saraswat N et al. Patient Controlled Epidural Analgesia during Labour: Effect of Addition of Background Infusion on Quality of Analgesia & Maternal Satisfaction. Indian J Anaesth 2009;53(6):649-53.

56. Halpern SH, Carvalho B. Patient-controlled epidural analgesia for labor. Anesth Analg 2009;108(3):921-8.

57. Sng BL, Sia AT, Lim Y, Woo D, Ocampo C. Comparison of computer-integrated patient-controlled epidural analgesia and patient-controlled epidural analgesia with a basal infusion for labour and delivery. Anaesth Intensive Care 2009;37(1):46-53.

58. Chen YM, Li Z, Wang AJ, Wang JM. Effect of labor analgesia with ropivacaine on the lactation of paturients. Zhonghua Fu Chan Ke Za Zhi 2008;43(7):502-5.

59. Lee HL, Lo LM, Chou CC, Chuah EC. Comparison between 0.08% ropivacaine and 0.06% levobupivacaine for epidural analgesia during nulliparous labor: a retrospective study in a single center. Chang Gung Med J 2011;34(3):286-92.

60. Liu EH, Sia AT. Rates of caesarean section and instrumental vaginal delivery in nulliparous women after low concentration epidural infusions or opioid analgesia: systematic review. BMJ 2004;328:1410-5.

61. Jorgensen H, Fomsgaard JS, Dirks J, Weterslev J, Andersoon B, Dahl JB. Effect of epidural bupivacaine vs combined epidural bupivacaine and morphine on gastrointestinal function and pain after major gynaecological surgery. Br J Anesth 2001;87(5):727-32.

62. Roelants F, Mercier-Fuzier V, Lavandhomme P. The effect of lidokaine test dose on analgesia and mobility after an epidural combination of neostigmine and sufentanil in early labor. Anesth Analg 2006;103(6):1534-9.

63. Balaji P, Dhillon P, Russell IF. Low-dose epidural top up for emergency caesarean delivery: a randomised comparison of levobupivacaine versus lidocaine /epinephrine /fentanyl. Int J Obstet Anesth 2009;18(4):335-41.

64. Segado Jiménez MI, Arias Delgado J, Domínguez Hervella F, Casas García ML, López Pérez A, Izquierdo Gutiérrez C. Epidural analgesia in

obstetrics: is there an effect on labor and delivery? Rev Esp Anesthesiol Reanim 2011;58(1):11-6.

65. Beilin Y, Mungall D, Hossain S, Bodian CA. Labor pain at the time of epidural analgesia and mode of delivery in nulliparous women presenting for an induction of labor. Obstet Gynecol 2009;114(4):764-9.

66. Aneiros F, Vazquez M, Valiño C, Taboada M, Sabaté S, Otero P et al. Does epidural versus combined spinal-epidural analgesia prolong labor and increase the risk of instrumental and cesarean delivery in nulliparous women? J Clin Anesth 2009;21(2):94-7.

67. Zimmer EZ, Jakobi P, Itskovitz-Eldor J, Weizman B, Solt I, Glik A et al. Adverse effects of epidural analgesia in labor. Eur J Obstet Gynaecol 2000;89:153-7.

68. Sienko J, Czajkowski K, Swiatek-Zdziencka M, Krawczynska-Wichrzycka R. Epidural analgesia and the course of delivery in term primiparas. Ginekol Pol 2005;76:806-11.

69. Harkins J, Carvalho B, Evers A, Mehta S, Riley ET. Survey of the Factors Associated with a Woman's Choice to Have an Epidural for Labor Analgesia. Anesthesiol Res Pract 2010;2010:ID 356789.

70. Fyneface-Ogan S, Mato CN, Anya SE. Epidural anesthesia: views and outcomes of women in labor in a Nigerian hospital. Ann Afr Med 2009;8(4):250-6.

71. Fanning RA, Briggs LP, Carey MF. Epidural analgesia practices for labour: results of a 2005 national survey in Ireland. Eur J Anaesthesiol 2009;26(3):235-44.

72. Burnstein R, Buckland R, Pickett JA. A survey of epidural analgesia for labour in the United Kingdom. Anesteshia 1999;54:634-40.

73. Weiniger CF, Ivri S, Ioscovich A, Grimberg L, Evron S, Ginosar Y. Obstetric anesthesia units in Israel: a national questionnaire-based survey. Int J Obstet Anesth 2010;19(4):410-6.

74. Panni MK. Labor pain at the time of epidural analgesia and mode of delivery in nulliparous women presenting for an induction of labor. Obstet Gynecol 2010;115(3):661.

75. Weigl W, Szymusik I, Borowska-Solonynko A, Kosińska-Kaczyńska K, Mayzner-Zawadzka E, Bomba-Opoń D et al. The influence of epidural analgesia on the course of labor. Ginekol Pol 2010;81(1):41-5.

76. Young P, Emery NC, Reisin R. Epidural analgesia for labor and delivery. N Engl J Med 2010;363(4):395.

77. Koppel BS, Chiechi M. Epidural analgesia for labor and delivery. N Engl J Med 2010;363(4):394-5.

78. Shokry M, Manaa EM, Shoukry RA, Shokeir MH, Elsedfy GO, Abd El-Aziz Ael-S. Effects of intrapartum epidural analgesia at high altitudes: maternal, fetal, and neonatal outcomes. A randomized controlled trial of two formulations of analgesics. Acta Obstet Gynecol Scand 2010;89(7):909-15.

79. Traynor JD, Dooley SL, Seyb S, Wong CA, Shadron A. Is management of epidural analgesia associated with an increased risk of cesarean delivery? Am J Obstet Gynecol 2000;182:1058-62.

80. Murphy DJ. Failure to progress in the second stage of labour. Curr Opin Obstet Gynecol 2001;13:557-61.

81. ACOG Committee Opinion No 269. Analgesia and Cesarean delivery rates. Obstet Gynecol 2002;99:369-70.

82. Frenea S, Chirossel C, Rodriguez R, Baguet JP, Racinet C, Payen JF. The effects of prolonged ambulation on labor with epidural analgesia. Anesth Analg 2004;98:224-9.

83. Nguyen US, Rothman KJ, Demissie S, Jackson DJ, Lang JM, Ecker JL. Epidural analgesia and risks of cesarean and operative vaginal deliveries in nulliparous and multiparous women. Matern Child Health J 2010;14(5):705-12.

84. Halpern SH, Abdallah FW. Effect of labor analgesia on labor outcome. Curr Opin Anaesthesiol 2010;23(3):317-22.

85. Schytt E, Waldenström U. Epidural analgesia for labor pain: whose choice? Acta Obstet Gynecol Scand 2010;89(2):238-42.

86. Bakhamees H, Hegazy E. Does epidural increase the incidence of cesarean delivery or instrumental labor in Saudi population? Middle East J Anesthesiol 2007;19(3):693-704.

87. Wang F, Shen X, Guo X, Peng Y, Gu X. Epidural analgesia in the latent phase of labor and risk of cesarean delivery: a five-year randomized controlled trial. Anesthesiology 2009;111(4):871-80.

88. Indraccolo U, Di Filippo D, Di Iorio R, Marinoni E, Roselli D, Indraccolo SR. Effect of epidural analgesia on operative vaginal birth rate. Clin Exp Obstet Gynecol 2011;38(3):221-4.

89. Wassen MM, Zuijlen J, Roumen FJ, Smits LJ, Marcus MA, Nijhuis JG. Early versus late epidural analgesia and risk of instrumental delivery in nulliparous women: a systematic review. BJOG 2011;118(6):655-61.

90. Eriksen LM, Nohr EA, Kjaergaard H. Mode of delivery after epidural analgesia in a cohort of low-risk nulliparas. Birth 2011;38(4):317-26.

91. Torvaldsen S, Roberts CL. No increased risk of caesarean or instrumental delivery for nulliparous women who have epidural analgesia early in (term) labour. Evid Based Med 2012;17(1):21-2.

92. Shahram N. Effects of epidural lidocaine analgesia on labor and delivery: A randomized prospective controlled trial. BMC Anesthesiol 2006;6:15.

93. Bruera E, Kim HN. Cancer pain. JAMA 2003;290:2476-93.

94. Gerli S, Favilli A, Acanfora MM, Bini V, Giorgini C, Di Renzo GC. Effect of epidural analgesia on labor and delivery: a retrospective study. J Matern Fetal Neonatal Med 2011;24(3):458-60.

95. Ekéus C, Cnattingius S, Hjern A. Epidural analgesia during labor among immigrant women in Sweden. Acta Obstet Gynecol Scand 2010;89(2):243-9.

96. Indraccolo U, Calabrese S, Di Iorio R, Corosu L, Marinoni E, Indraccolo SR. Impact of the medicalization of labor on mode of delivery. Clin Exp Obstet Gynecol 2010;37(4):273-7.

97. Mayberry LJ, Clemmens D, Anindya D. Epidural analgesia side effects, co-interventions and care of women during childbirth: A systematic review. Am J Obstet Gynecol 2002; 186(5):81-93.

98. Lieberman E, O'Donoghue C. Unintended effects of epidural analgesia during labor: A systematic review. Am J Obstet Gynecol 2002;186:31-68.

99. Nafisi S. Effects of epidural lidocaine analgesia on labor and delivery: a randomized, prospective controlled trial. BMC Anesthesiol 2006;16:15.

100. Caruselli M, Camilletti G, Torino G, Pizzi S, Amici M, Piattellini G et al. Epidural analgesia during labor and incidence of cesarian section: prospective study. J Matern Fetal Neonatal Med 2011;24(2):250-2.

101. Lee S, Lew E, Lim Y, Sia AT. Failure of augmentation of labor epidural analgesia for intrapartum cesarean delivey: a retrospective review. Anesth Analg 2009;108:252-4.

102. Fratelli N, Prefumo F, Andrico S, Lorandi A, Recupero D, Tomasoni G et al. Effects of epidural analgesia on uterine artery Doppler in labour. Br J Anaesth 2011;106(2):221-4.

103. Lee N-J, Sim J, Lee MS, Ahn W, Han SS, Lee HM. A survey on informed consent process for epidural analgesia in labor pain in Korea. Korean J Anesthesiol 2010;59:34-8.

104. Chichester ML, Hoffman MK, Colmorgen GH, Shlossman PA. Labor analgesia for patients with preterm premature rupture of membranes. J Perinatol 2010;30(10):650-4.

105. Ekéus C, Hjern A, Hjelmstedt A. The need for epidural analgesia is related to birthweight – a population-based register study. Acta Obstet Gynecol Scand 2009;88(4):397-401.

106. El-Kerdawy H, Farouk A. Labor analgesia in preeclampsia: remifentanil patient controlled intravenous analgesia versus epidural analgesia. Middle East J Anesthesiol 2010;20(4):539-45.

107. Malvasi A, Tinelli A, Brizzi A, Greco F, Celleno D, Tinelli R. Long-term epidural analgesia treatment in pre-eclamptic women: a preliminary trial. J Obstet Gynaecol 2009;29(2):114-8.

108. Roofthooft E. Anesthesia for the morbidly obese parturient. Curr Opin Anaesthesiol 2009;22(3):341-6.

109. Sidelnick C, Karmon A, Levy A, Greemberg L, Shapira Y, Sheiner E. Intra-partum epidural analgesia in grandmultiparous women. J Matern Fetal Neonatal Med 2009;22(4):348-52.

110. Campbell DC, Tran T. Conversion of epidural labour analgesia to epidural anesthesia for intrapartum Cesarean delivery. Can J Anaesth 2009;56(1):19-26.

111. Hillyard SG, Bate TE, Corcoran TB, Paech MJ, O'Sullivan G. Extending epidural analgesia for emergency Caesarean section: a meta-analysis. Br J Anaesth 2011;107(5):668-78.

112. Lao HC, Hseu SS, Huang CJ, Chan KH, Kuo CD. The effect of heart rate variability on request for labour epidural analgesia. Anaesthesia 2009;64(8):856-62.

113. Atanasova M, Nikolov A. Epidural analgesia for vaginal delivery. Influence over the delivery, fetal presentation, the method of delivery and lactation. Akush Ginekol 2011;50(6):28-36.

114. Martino V, Iliceto N, Simeoni U. Occipitoposterior fetal head position, maternal and neonatal outcome. Minerva Gynecol 2007;59:459-64.

115. Gillesby E, Burns S, Dempsey A, Kirby S, Mogensen K, Naylor K et al.. Comparison of delayed versus immediate pushing during second stage of labor for nulliparous women with epidural anesthesia. J Obstet Gynecol Neonatal Nurs 2010;39(6):635-44.

116. Kelly M, Johnson E, Lee V, Massey L, Purser D, Ring K, Sanderson S et al. Delayed versus immediate pushing in second stage of labor. MCN Am J Matern Child Nurs 2010;35(2):81-8.

117. Le Ray C, Audibert F, Goffinet F, Fraser W. When to stop pushing: effects of duration of second-stage expulsion efforts on maternal and neonatal outcomes in nulliparous women with epidural analgesia. Am J Obstet Gynecol 2009;201(4):361-7.

118. Cooper GM, MacArthur C, Wilson MJ, Moore PA, Shennan A; COMET Study Group UK. Satisfaction, control and pain relief: short- and long-term assessments in a randomised controlled trial of low-dose and traditional epidurals and a non-epidural comparison group. Int J Obstet Anesth 2010;19(1):31-7.

119. Liang MY, Pagel PS. Bilateral interhemispheric subdural hematoma after inadvertent lumbar puncture in a parturient. Can J Anaesth 2012;59(4):389-93.

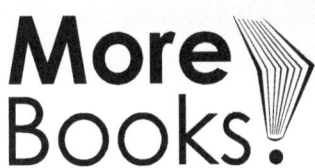
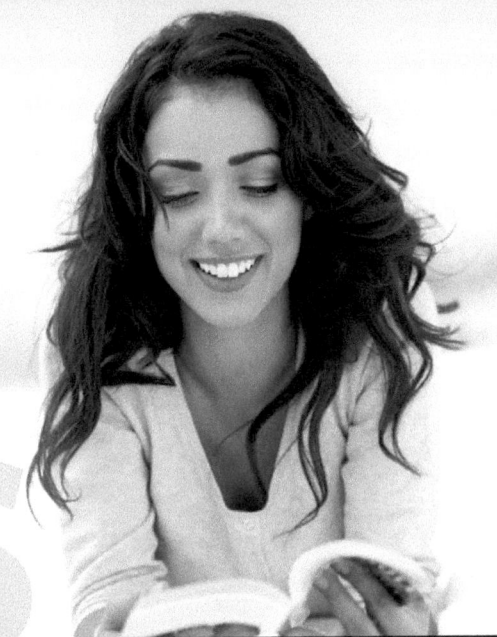
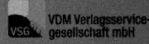

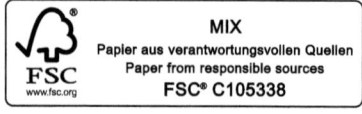